PALEO SMOOTHIES RECIPES JUMPSTART COOKBOOK

Over 50 Mouthwatering Recipes

Ready In 10 Minutes;

Lose the Weight & Find Your Path Back to Health

SARAH MOORE

SARAH MOORE

ISBN: 9781549674273

CONTENTS

INTRODUCTION

Congratulations for choosing *Paleo Smoothies Recipes*, these recipes helps you to lose weight, gain health, detox without losing energy and vitality. Coming to the facts, there are so many different types of benefits of paleo smoothies, but due to lack of awareness, people are missing safe way to maintain healthy long life.

There are a number of ways to make delicious and nutritious paleo smoothies than simply adding bunches of ingredients willy-nilly. So, to avoid this, in the following chapters will discuss each and every step to getting started with paleo smoothies including health benefits and nutritional information.

Additionally, you will learn different types of helpful tricks and tips to ensure your paleo smoothie's habit develops as quickly and easily as possible, including how to processed with existing blender to avoid cost before you are fully committed to follow the diet.

After that you will find 25 fruit smoothies and 25 vegetable smoothies regardless if you are interested to prepare them to lose weight, detoxify and boost health with increasing energy and vitality. This recipe's ensures that you will definitely gain energy in less time period without losing your health.

The key to successfully starting a new habit is doing everything what you can do within your power with strong mind and dedication to improve your health by following our diet, some of the successful habit formations are reminder, routine and reward yourself with additional juice when you achieved your weekly goal and remind yourself about wonderful benefits.

CHAPTER 1: ABOUT PALEO SMOOTHIES

The PALEO Smoothies are one of the most healthiest ways you can eat in light of the fact that it is one of the nutritious methodologies that works with your hereditary qualities to enable you to remain lean, solid and vigorous. The smoothies are one the best way to integrate a large amount of nutrition's as required to reduce body weight, far more than you could get by eating fruits and veggies alone. Fruit and Vegetable smoothies are packed with full of leafy plants, fruits and water with delicious taste and also helpful in reducing cravings, boosting the immune system, increasing energy levels with vitality and assisting in weight loss.

Easy to digest: The fruits and vegetables contain more valuable nutrients than any other food items and less time to digest, this is because body spends, the more effort of energy in the digestion process so your body doesn't have to. These smoothies contain high quantity of *phytonutrients,* which keeps your digestive system functioning properly and improves health with reducing future diseases.

Great way to start the day: Paleo smoothies allows you to consume more amount of vitamins and nutrients then dosage you get from vegetables and fruits per servings, greens will give super charging energy if you are starting out the day or midafternoon boost to get you through the rest of the work day.

Highly portable: Smoothies can be prepared in less time (5-10 minutes) and makes your dream come true, which can be stored for a long time in a cool place but immediate consumption will give best results.

Great option to replace a meal: When you think about meal replacement, one of the best and great option is smoothies, which are homemade and also low calorie delicious shakes, packed with protein and fiber, which makes you don't eat junk food in between meals.

I can explain most numerous health benefits of paleo smoothies, but you are going to learn more information as we go through this book and you will discover excellent health benefits yourself, once again thank you for downloading the book and enjoy each and every recipe you encounter and this book makes you to make your own recipes for good health.

CHAPTER 2: WHY PALEO SMOOTHIES

Research in science, natural chemistry, ophthalmology, dermatology and numerous different other agencies says that paleo diet is modern diet with full of nutrients, which are essentially required for body. Paleo helps to reduce some the diseases like degenerative diseases, obesity, cancer, diabetes, heart disease, digestive problems, alzheimer's, coronary illness, depression, infertility and also helps in different ways, as mentioned below:

Weight loss: After trying paleo smoothies, you will be surprised to learn that smoothies are one of the best ways to lose weight without any difficultly because this recipe's contains high quantity of water filled with green leafy veggies and fruits with high fiber content, which helps you stay full for a long time and also reduce cravings for junk food.

Rich nutrients: When we cook any food for a long time in high temperature, it will destroy many nutrients, but in case of smoothies all ingredients are raw and full loaded with vitamins, minerals, antioxidants, water, fiber, phytonutrients, anti-inflammatory substances and chlorophyll. This chlorophyll has a similar structure to hemoglobin in blood, which act as cleansing blood transfusion.

Detoxification: Normally our body tries to eliminate toxins from our body, but due to lack of organic food, it will slow down the body's detoxification system and causes weight gain, we have to thank to paleo smoothies because it will produce fiber, which helps you in cleansing your digestive system and eliminate toxins.

Anti-aging: When you start drinking paleo smoothies, you can see changes not only inside but also outside of the body, especially after toxin free slowly it will start eliminating wrinkles, acne and dark circles under eye and makes your face young again.

Hydration: Normally, staying hydrated gives energy and helps your brain, immune system and digestive system work properly without any defects. Simple way to check yourself whether you are hydrated or dehydrated by looking at your urine color, if it is strong yellow color, then you are dehydrated that means our body directly saying that we forgot to drink sufficient water due to our busy work, in this case we have to thank paleo smoothies because it contains 70% of required water and avoids us from dehydration, now you will start realizing the advantages of smoothies in your life.

CHAPTER 3: TIPS AND TRICKS TO MAKE
DELICIOUS SMOOTHIES

Why smoothies: Smoothies allows easy absorption of nutrients straight into the bloodstream and helps to heal the body and digestive system very fast and aids in weight control but smoothies have pulp which slow down the digestive system.

Pre-prepare your ingredients: Depending on your next day timetable you can prepare required ingredients in advance to avoid last movement confusions and also you can make right smoothie depending on your diet (weight loss, energy and vitality or detox).

Fresh smoothies: Most people will think about frozen food, but remember fresh greens are always going to be healthier than frozen items. Prepare them first and freeze them until you are ready to use it, this will be the best way to use and keep your body healthier.

Get started with an existing mixer: If you are interested getting started creating delicious and nutritious paleo smoothies, at first no need to spend $300 or more on a mixer before you figure out that green juices are really working for you, it's important that you dice, chop and shred all your ingredients as needed for perfect pure smoothie and also secure motor of the mixer. The best way to secure mixer motor is, start on slower speeds and gradually increase speed to next option every 20 seconds or so.

Protein myth: Paleo smoothie contain 30 to 40 percent of greens are a great source of protein in the body, which provide protein in the form of amino acids and building blocks of protein. This makes body to utilize them easier than other animal products and easier for the digestive system.

If you feel that you required additional protein for your body due to heavy workouts, feel free to add protein powder in your mixer while making paleo smoothie.

Basic step: Begin each day with a few glasses of water and followed by a cup of detox tea with natural sweetener which will provide cleansing support for your kidneys and liver and helps to flush away toxins from the body.

CHAPTER 4: LIST OF PALEO FOOD

Why vegetables and fruits?

Eating vegetables and natural products as a major aspect of our day by day life will help to overcome some genuine medical issues. Most fruits and vegetables are normally low in fat and calories.

Fruits and vegetables will have some similar nutrients, micronutrients are a class of supplements that incorporate vitamins, minerals and phytonutrients that are essential for body to maintain proper healthy functioning of the organs.

Leafy vegetables have more micronutrients than any other vegetables or fruits like iron, calcium and magnesium. Which play key role in the proper functioning of the nervous system as well as the immune system.

Root vegetables are the powerhouses of minerals, vitamins and also additionally supply carbohydrates, especially complex-carbohydrates, which gradually supply constant energy to the body.

Basically, fruits have low fat and more fiber and water, this make digestive system healthy because fruits have low sodium-content with natural sugar.

VEGETABLES	Celery, Tomatoes, Bell Peppers, Onions, Leeks, Kohlrabi, Green Onions, Eggplants, Cauliflower, Broccoli, Asparagus, Cucumber, Cabbage, Brussels Sprouts, Artichokes, Okra, Avocados
GREEN LEAFY VEG	Lettuce, Spinach, Collard Greens, Kale, Beet Top, Mustard Greens, Dandelion, Swiss Chard, Watercress, Turnip Greens, Seaweeds, Endive, Arugula (Rocket), Bok Choy, Rapini, Chicory, Radicchio
ROOT VEGETABLES	Carrots, Beets, Turnips, Parsnips, Rutabaga, Sweet Potatoes, Radish, Jerusalem Artichokes, Yams, Cassava
WINTER SQUASH	Butternut Squash, Spaghetti Squash Acorn Squash, Pumpkin, Buttercup Squash.
SUMMER SQUASH	Zucchini, Yellow Summer Squash, Yellow Crookneck Squash
FRUIT	Bananas, Apples, Oranges, Berries (Strawberry, Cranberry, Blueberry, Blackberry, Raspberry), Plantains, Grapefruit, Pears, Peaches, Nectarines, Plums, Pomegranates, Pineapple, Papaya, Grapes, Cantaloupe, Cherries, Apricot, Watermelon, Honeydew Melon, Kiwi, Lemon, Lime, Lychee, Mango, Tangerine, Coconut, Figs, Dates, Olives, Passion Fruit, Persimmon
NUTS & SEEDS	Pistachios, Brazil Nuts, Sunflower Seeds, Sesame Seeds, Chia Seeds, Flax Seeds, Pumpkin Seeds (Pepitas), Pecans, Walnuts, Pine Nuts, Macadamia Nuts, Chestnuts,

	Cashews, Almonds, Hazelnuts
HERBS	Parsley, Thyme, Lavender, Mint, Basil, Rosemary, Chives, Tarragon, Oregano, Sage, Dill, Bay Leaves, Coriander
SPICES & OTHERS	Ginger, Garlic, Onions, Black Pepper, Hot Peppers, Star Anise, Fennel Seeds, Mustard Seeds, Cayenne Pepper, Cumin, Turmeric, Cinnamon, Nutmeg, Paprika, Vanilla, Cloves, Chilies, Horseradish

CHAPTER 5: LIST OF PALEO FOOD TO AVOID

Why Sugar is bad?

The vast majority of us consider "sugar" for coffee or espresso, but in natural terms, sugar is only the building blocks of carbohydrates in body. Research studies say that sugar and weight gain is tremendous. Sugar is the one of the main cause of every modern health problem.

- Sugar must be used by the liver and can't be utilized for vitality by your body's cells, similar effects on the liver as alcohol.

- Sugar reacts with proteins and fats in our bodies 7 times more than glucose.

- Sugar increases uric acid production in body, which causes kidney stones.

- Abundance sugar alone can cause every one of the issues related with the metabolic disorder (heart disease, obesity, diabetes).

DAIRY	Milk, Butter, Buttermilk, Yogurt, Kefir, Cream, Ghee, Ice Cream, Powdered Milk, Cottage Cheese, Everything Came From Animal's Teat
SUGAR	Avoid Sugar (Try Artificial Sweeteners)
PROCESSED FOOD	Frozen Meals, Fast Food, Sweets
ALCOHOL	Everything

CHAPTER 6: 26 MOUTHWATERING FRUIT SMOOTHIES

Recipe 1: Banana Hemp Seed Smoothie

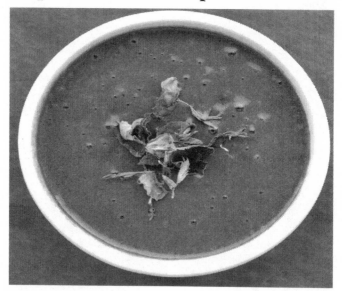

Ingredients

- Bananas 2
- Frozen peach slices 1 cup
- Almond butter 2 tbsp.
- Hemp seeds 1 tbsp.
- Dry rose and lavender petals 4
- Water 2 cups

Preparation Method

1. In a blender, place all ingredients expect dry rose and lavender petals and blend on medium speed or until smooth.
2. Pour into serving glass, garnish with dry rose and lavender petals and enjoy the taste.Nutritional Information

Preparation Time:10 minutes

- Servings per Recipe: 2
- Calories: 250
- Protein: 5.4g
- Fat: 12g
- Carbohydrates: 34.9g

Benefits

- Banana reduces risk of heart diseases due to its powerful antioxidants
- Due to its more antioxidants, helps to improve immunity function and reduce inflammation
- Peaches have potassium, helps to proper nerve signaling and cellular functions
- Hemp seeds help to reduce cholesterol and blood pressure

Recipe 2: Appe Berry Smoothie

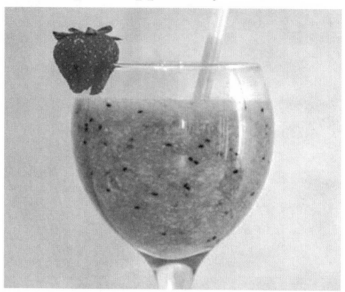

Ingredients

- Green apple 4 oz.
- Chia seeds 1 tbsp.
- Raspberries 4 oz.
- Fig 2 oz.
- Lemon juice 1 tbsp.

Preparation Method

1. In a blender, place all ingredients and blend on medium speed or until smooth.
2. Pour into serving glass and enjoy the taste.

Nutritional Information

- Preparation Time: 10 minutes
- Servings per Recipe: 2
- Calories: 190
- Protein: 2.9g
- Fat: 1.7g
- Carbohydrates: 19g

Benefits

- Apple is stuffed with vitamins helps in premature aging
- Chia seeds help to boost your metabolism
- Raspberries helps in memory improvement
- Fig helps to control blood pressure
- Lemon helps to lose weight

Recipe 3: Melon Smoothie

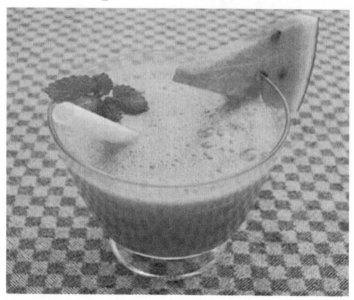

Ingredients

- Watermelon 5.5 oz.
- Banana 3.5 oz.
- Cilantro 3.5 oz.
- Lemon 1 oz.
- Wheatgrass 1 tbsp.
- Dates 2 pieces

Preparation Method

1. In a blender, place all ingredients and blend on medium speed or until smooth.
2. Pour into serving glass and enjoy the taste.

Nutritional Information

- Preparation Time: 10 minutes
- Servings per Recipe: 2
- Calories: 240
- Protein: 7.7g
- Fat: 0.71g

- Carbohydrates: 16.6g

Benefits

- Watermelon works as a natural Viagra, which relaxes and dilates blood vessels in the body
- Banana reduces risk of heart diseases due to its powerful antioxidants
- Cilantro helps to build strong bones and also known as anti-diabetic plant
- Wheat grass used to neutralize toxins in the body
- Dates helps to reduce weight

Recipe 4: Ginger Grape Smoothie

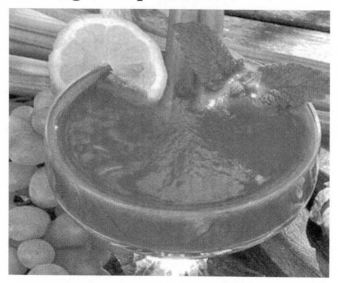

Ingredients

- Seedless grapes 3.5 oz.
- Ginger 1 oz.
- Ground chia seed 1 ½ tbsp.
- Cayenne Pepper 2 tsp.
- Sage 1 tbsp.

Preparation Method

1. In a blender, place all ingredients and blend on medium speed or until smooth.
2. Pour into serving glass and enjoy the taste.

Nutritional Information

- Preparation Time: 8 minutes
- Servings per Recipe: 1
- Calories: 206
- Protein: 5.2g
- Fat: 3.3g
- Carbohydrates: 13.5g

Benefits

- Grapes helps to boost the immune system
- Ginger prevents morning sickness
- Chia seeds and pepper help to boost your metabolism
- Sage helps to improve digestive system

Recipe 5: Lingo Pomegranate Smoothie

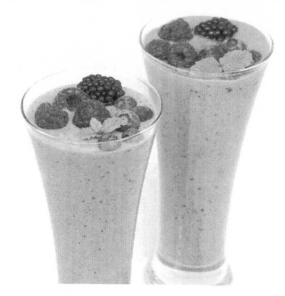

Ingredients

- Pomegranate juice 1 ½ cup
- Water 1 cup
- Mixed berries 2 cups
- Thyme 2 tbsp.
- Lingonberries 1 oz.
- Ground flax seeds 1 tbsp.

Preparation Method

1. In a blender, place all ingredients and blend on medium speed or until smooth.
2. Pour into serving glass and enjoy the taste.

Nutritional Information

- Preparation Time: 10 minutes
- Servings per Recipe: 2
- Calories: 189
- Protein: 3g
- Fat: 1.6g

- Carbohydrates: 26g

Benefits

- Pomegranate helps to keep diabetes in control
- Berries boosts the immune system and flu protection
- Thyme is a natural remedy for bronchitis and cough
- Lingo berry contain high amounts of arbutin, helps to reduce age spots
- Flaxseed is protective effect against breast cancer, prostate cancer, and colon cancer

Recipe 6: Summer Sweet Smoothie

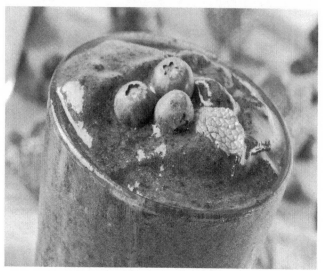

Ingredients

- Cranberry juice 2 cups
- Strawberries 1 ½ cup
- Blueberries ¾ cup
- Watermelon 5 oz.
- Banana 1
- Fresh fig 2
- Flax seeds 1 tbsp.
- Wheat germ 1 tbsp.

Preparation Method

1. In a blender, place all ingredients and blend on medium speed or until smooth.
2. Pour into serving glass and enjoy the taste.

Nutritional Information

- Preparation Time: 10 minutes
- Servings per Recipe: 2
- Calories: 190
- Protein: 4.1g
- Fat: 2.1g

- Carbohydrates: 19g

Benefits

- Cranberries help to treat urinary tract infections
- Watermelon works as a natural viagra, which relaxes and dilates blood vessels in the body
- Blueberries, due to its high antioxidants, it neutralizes most of the free radicals that cause damage to DNA
- Strawberry acts like immune booster
- Fig helps to control blood pressure
- Banana reduces risk of heart diseases
- Wheat germ increases energy

Recipe 7: Black forest Smoothie

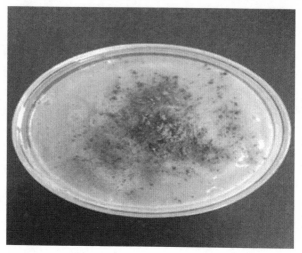

Ingredients

- Orange juice 1 ½ cup
- Almond yogurt 1 tbsp.
- Dates 5 pieces
- Frozen forest fruits 1 ½ cup

Preparation Method

1. In a blender, place all ingredients and blend on medium speed or until smooth.
2. Pour into serving glass and enjoy the taste.

Nutritional Information

- Preparation Time: 5 minutes
- Servings per Recipe: 1
- Calories: 183
- Protein: 3.6g
- Fat: 2.3g
- Carbohydrates: 20g

Benefits

- Orange protect the skin from radical damage

- Dates helps to reduce weight
- Almond yogurt provide healthy fat for heart

Recipe 8: Aprines Smoothie

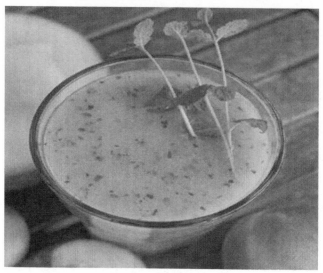

Ingredients

- Ginger root 1 oz.
- Cinnamon 1 tbsp.
- Water 1 cup
- Nectarines 3.5 oz.
- Apricot 2 oz.

Preparation Method

1. In a blender, place all ingredients and blend on medium speed or until smooth.
2. Pour into serving glass and enjoy the taste.

Nutritional Information

- Preparation Time: 10 minutes
- Servings per Recipe: 1
- Calories: 147
- Protein: 5.1g
- Fat: 0.9g
- Carbohydrates: 18g

Benefits

- Ginger produces sexual arousal, which increases stimulation in the brain
- Cinnamon helps to lose weight faster
- Nectarines help to build and maintain healthy teeth, skin, tissue (soft and bone) and mucus membranes
- Apricot is rich in vitamins and minerals. Helps to get relief from earaches

Recipe 9: Granny Smooth Smoothie

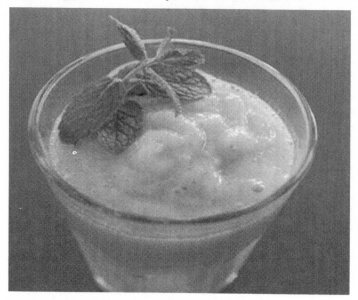

Ingredients

- Plantains 5
- Granny smith apple 3.5 oz.
- Avocado 1 oz.
- Jicama 1 oz.
- Cilantro 2 tsp.
- Lime 1 tbsp.
- Hemp 1 tbsp.
- Medjool date 1
- Water (max to line)

Preparation Method

- In a blender, place all ingredients and blend on medium speed or until smooth.
- Pour into serving glass and enjoy the taste.

Nutritional Information

- Preparation Time: 10 minutes

- Servings per Recipe: 1
- Calories: 214
- Protein: 5.3g
- Fat: 9g
- Carbohydrates: 31g

Benefits

- Plantains helps to prevent dry eyes, eye infection and unhealthy skin
- Avocado helps to reduce belly fat
- Jicama helps to increase bone strength and functionalities of brain
- Cilantro helps to build strong bones and also known as anti-diabetic plant
- Hemp seeds help to reduce cholesterol and blood pressure

Recipe 10: Papaya Belly Smoothie

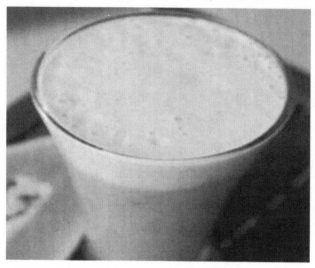

Ingredients

- Papaya 6.5 oz.
- Coconut water 1 cup
- Lime juice 4 tsp.
- Dates 5

Preparation Method

1. In a blender, place all ingredients and blend on medium speed or until smooth.
2. Pour into serving glass and enjoy the taste.

Nutritional Information

- Preparation Time: 10 minutes
- Servings per Recipe: 1
- Calories: 201
- Protein: 2.7g
- Fat: 1.1g
- Carbohydrates: 16g

Benefits

- Coconut water helps to boost metabolism of the body
- Lime helps to prevent respiratory problems
- Papaya helps to prevent infections (kills intestine worms) and relieves toothache

Recipe 11: Melon Smoothie

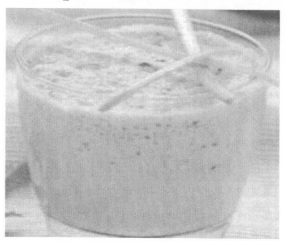

Ingredients

- Honeydew Melon 4 oz.
- Coconut flakes 1 oz.
- Mint 3 leaves
- Strawberries 2 oz.
- Cinnamon ½ tsp.
- Almond milk 1 cup
- Coconut water 1 cup

Preparation Method

1. In a blender, place all ingredients and blend on medium speed or until smooth.
2. Pour into serving glass and enjoy the taste.

Nutritional Information

- Preparation Time: 10 minutes
- Servings per Recipe: 2
- Calories: 376
- Protein: 10.9g
- Fat: 15g
- Carbohydrates: 29g

Benefits

- Mint is a great palate cleanser, promotes effective digestion
- Ground Cinnamon protect the body from oxidative damage caused by free radicals and reduces DNA damage
- Honey melons improves blood pressure levels and repairs tissues in the body
- Strawberry acts like immune booster

Recipe 12: Papaya Detox

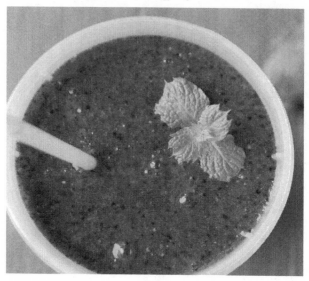

Ingredients

- Passion fruit 2 oz.
- Papaya 3.5 oz.
- Plums 3.5 oz.
- Ginger 1 oz.
- Lemon juice 1 oz.
- Lavender 1 tsp.
- Coconut water (to max line)

Preparation Method

1. In a blender, place all ingredients and blend on medium speed or until smooth.
2. Pour into serving glass and enjoy the taste.

Nutritional Information

- Preparation Time: 10 minutes
- Servings per Recipe: 1
- Calories: 166
- Protein: 2.9g

- Fat: 6g
- Carbohydrates: 17.5g

Benefits

- Passion fruit, due to it's high iron contains helps to improve blood circulation and also gives relief from asthma, insomnia and whopping cough
- Papaya helps to prevent infections (kills intestine worms) and relieves toothache
- Plums fight obesity and best for diabetic patience's (reduces triglyceride and glucose in the body)
- Lavender helps to reduce anxiety and emotional stress

Recipe 13: Creamer Smoothie

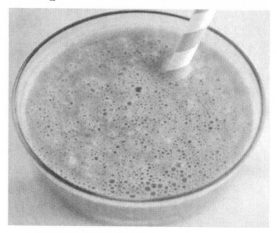

Ingredients

- Frozen mango 1 cup
- Almond milk 1 cup
- Ice cubes 2
- Tangerine 2 oz.
- Orange juice 1 cup
- Peach juice 1 cup
- Peach yogurt 2 oz.

Preparation Method

1. In a blender, place all ingredients and blend on medium speed or until smooth.
2. Pour into serving glass and enjoy the taste.

Nutritional Information

- Preparation Time: 10 minutes
- Servings per Recipe: 1
- Calories: 156
- Protein: 2.8g
- Fat: 2g
- Carbohydrates: 18.8g

Benefits

- Mango boosts immune system
- Tangerine helps to cure sepsis, cuts and wounds
- Peaches have potassium, helps to proper nerve signaling and cellular functions

Recipe 14: Pineapple Smoothie

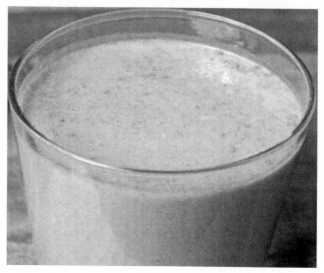

Ingredients

- Banana 1
- Oranges 2
- Lemon 1 oz.
- Fresh ginger 1 tbsp.
- Chia seeds 1 oz.
- Pine apple 2 ½ cup
- Water ½ cup

Preparation Method

- In a blender, place all ingredients and blend on medium speed or until smooth.
- Pour into serving glass and enjoy the taste.

Nutritional Information

- Preparation Time: 10 minutes
- Servings per Recipe: 2
- Calories: 369
- Protein: 9g
- Fat: 5.5g

- Carbohydrates: 19.1g

Benefits

- Banana reduces risk of heart diseases due to its powerful antioxidants
- Orange protect the skin from radical damage
- Lemon juice to a beverage will help increase weight loss
- Chia seeds help to boost your metabolism
- Pineapple helps to increase energy and decreases risk of diseases

Recipe 15: Fuji Olives Smoothie

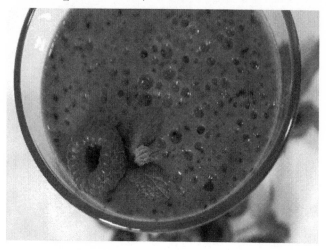

Ingredients

- Coconut water 1 cup
- Fuji apple 1
- Pear 1
- Shaved coconut 1 tbsp.
- Olives 4 pieces
- Raspberry 2 oz.

Preparation Method

1. In a blender, place all ingredients and blend on medium speed or until smooth.
2. Pour into serving glass and enjoy the taste.

Nutritional Information

- Preparation Time: 10 minutes
- Servings per Recipe: 1
- Calories: 348
- Protein: 15.1g
- Fat: 4.2g
- Carbohydrates: 18.8g

Benefits

- Coconut water balances the electrolytes in the body which improves blood circulation and muscle function
- Pears are natural boost of energy because of its glucose and fructose
- Raspberries helps in memory improvement
- Olives protect against ulcers and colon
- Coconut flakes might lower your risk of heart disease, diabetes

Recipe 16: Chia Berry Smoothie

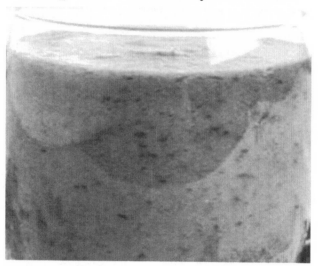

Ingredients

- Banana 1
- Blueberries 3 oz.
- Strawberries 1 oz.
- Cherries 1 oz.
- Chia seeds 1 tbsp.
- Almond milk 1 cup

Preparation Method

1. In a blender, place all ingredients and blend on medium speed or until smooth.
2. Pour into serving glass and enjoy the taste.

Nutritional Information

- Preparation Time: 10 minutes
- Servings per Recipe: 1
- Calories: 321
- Protein: 7.7g
- Fat: 6.1g
- Carbohydrates: 21.1g

Benefits

- Banana reduces risk of heart diseases due to its powerful antioxidants
- Blueberries, due to its high antioxidants, it neutralizes most of the free radicals that cause damage to DNA
- Chia seeds help to boost your metabolism
- Cherries helps to produce melatonin for healthy sleep and reduce muscle pain after some exercises
- Strawberry acts like immune booster

Recipe 17: Green Mango Smoothie

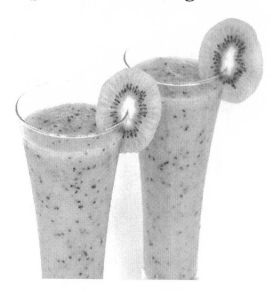

Ingredients

- Mango 5.5 oz.
- Lime 1 oz.
- Half Banana
- Kiwi 2 cups
- Coconut milk 1 cup

Preparation Method

1. In a blender, place all ingredients and blend on medium speed or until smooth.
2. Pour into serving glass and enjoy the taste.

Nutritional Information

- Preparation Time: 10 minutes
- Servings per Recipe: 1
- Calories: 318
- Protein: 10g
- Fat: 3.1g
- Carbohydrates: 19.9g

Benefits

- Mango boosts immune system
- Lime helps to prevent respiratory problems
- Kiwi is full of antioxidants, so it will help to prevent diseases
- Coconut milk consumption helps to protect the body from infections and viruses

Recipe 18: Herb Lychee Smoothie

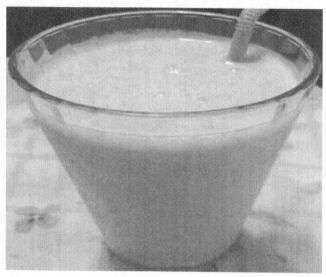

Ingredients

- Strawberries 6
- Basil leaves 6
- Chia seeds 1 oz.
- Banana 1
- Lychee 2 ½ cup
- Almond milk 1 cup

Preparation Method

1. In a blender, place all ingredients and blend on medium speed or until smooth.
2. Pour into serving glass and enjoy the taste.

Nutritional Information

- Preparation Time: 10 minutes
- Servings per Recipe: 1
- Calories: 266
- Protein: 7.2g
- Fat: 3.1g
- Carbohydrates: 22g

Benefits

- Basil prevent oxygen based damages
- Chia seeds help to boost your metabolism
- Lychee protect skin against harmful UV rays and beneficial for weight loss
- Banana reduces risk of heart diseases due to its powerful antioxidants
- Strawberry acts like immune booster

Recipe 19: Avocado Smoothie

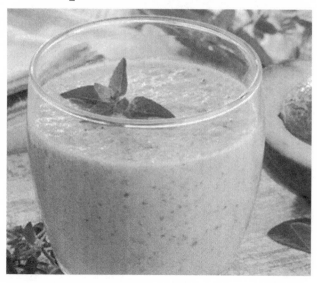

Ingredients

- Avocado 3 oz.
- Cranberry 3 oz.
- Lemon juice ½ cup
- Cinnamon 1 tsp.
- Water 1 cup

Preparation Method

- In a blender, place all ingredients and blend on medium speed or until smooth.
- Pour into serving glass and enjoy the taste.

Nutritional Information

- Preparation Time: 10 minutes
- Servings per Recipe: 1
- Calories: 224
- Protein: 15.1g
- Fat: 2.3g
- Carbohydrates: 16.9g

Benefits

- Avocado helps to reduce belly fat
- Lemon and cinnamon helps to lose weight faster
- Cranberries helps to treat urinary tract infections

Recipe 20: Max Mix Smoothie

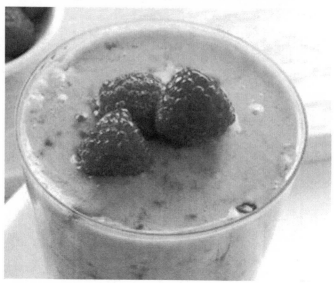

Ingredients

- Raspberries 3 oz.
- Pineapple 3 oz.
- Blueberries 3 oz.
- Strawberries2 cups
- Vanillas extract 2 tsp.
- Water 1 ½ cup
- Dates 3 pieces

Preparation Method

- In a blender, place all ingredients and blend on medium speed or until smooth.
- Pour into serving glass and enjoy the taste.

Nutritional Information

- Preparation Time: 10 minutes
- Servings per Recipe: 2
- Calories: 110.2
- Protein: 3.2g

- Fat: 1.4g
- Carbohydrates: 23.3g

Benefits

- Pineapple helps to increase energy and decreases risk of obesity
- Blueberries, due to its high antioxidants, it neutralizes most of the free radicals that cause damage to DNA
- Raspberries helps in memory improvement
- Dates helps to reduce weight

Recipe 21: Papaya Ginger Smoothie

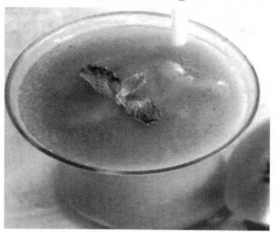

Ingredients

- Papaya 5.4 oz.
- Peach 2.5 oz.
- Pear 2.5 oz.
- Flax seeds 1 tbsp.
- Ginger 1 tsp.
- Fresh Mint 4 leaves
- Almond yogurt 2 oz.
- Ice cubes 4
- Water (to max line)

Preparation Method

1. In a blender, place all ingredients and blend on medium speed or until smooth.
2. Pour into serving glass and enjoy the taste.

Nutritional Information

- Preparation Time: 10 minutes
- Servings per Recipe: 1
- Calories: 278
- Protein: 3.9g
- Fat: 4.8g

- Carbohydrates: 21g

Benefits

- Papaya helps to prevent infections (kills intestine worms) and relieves toothache
- Flaxseed is protective effect against breast cancer, prostate cancer, and colon cancer
- Peaches have potassium, helps to proper nerve signaling and cellular functions
- Pears are natural boost of energy because of its glucose and fructose
- Mint is good for digestion, memory loss and prevent pimples

Recipe 22: Banan Melon Smoothie

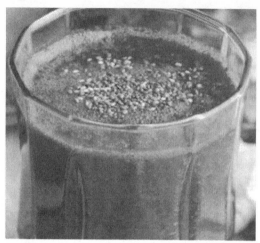

Ingredients

- Mixed berries 2.5 oz.
- Banana 1
- Ground hemp seeds 1 tbsp.
- Water 1 ½ cup
- Watermelon 1 oz.
- Almond milk 1 cup

Preparation Method

1. In a blender, place all ingredients and blend on medium speed or until smooth.
2. Pour into serving glass and enjoy the taste.

Nutritional Information

- Preparation Time: 10 minutes
- Servings per Recipe: 1
- Calories: 302
- Protein: 6.7g
- Fat: 5g
- Carbohydrates: 24.3g

Benefits

- Berries provide protection against the endothelial dysfunction
- Banana reduces risk of heart diseases
- Hemp seeds help to reduce cholesterol and blood pressure
- Watermelon works as a natural viagra, which relaxes and dilates blood vessels in the body

Recipe 23: Brain-Boosting Smoothie

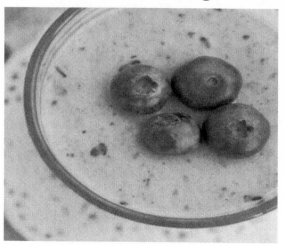

Ingredients

- Walnuts 6
- Banana 1
- Blueberries 3 oz.
- Almond milk 1 ½ cup
- Mango 2 oz.

Preparation Method

1. In a blender, place all ingredients and blend on medium speed or until smooth.
2. Pour into serving glass and enjoy the taste.

Nutritional Information

- Preparation Time: 10 minutes
- Servings per Recipe: 1
- Calories: 411
- Protein: 9.1g
- Fat: 4.9g
- Carbohydrates: 18g

Benefits

- Walnut reduce risk of excessive clotting and inflammation
- Blueberries, due to its high antioxidants, it neutralizes most of the free radicals that cause damage to DNA
- Mango boosts immune system

Recipe 24: Almond Chia Smoothie

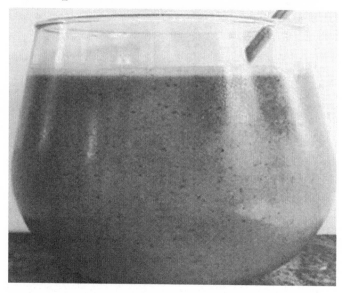

Ingredients

- Plums 3 cups
- Blueberries 2.5 oz.
- Strawberries 2 oz.
- Chia seeds 1 tbsp.
- Almonds 1 oz.
- Coconut water 1 cup
- Water ½ cup

Preparation Method

1. In a blender, place all ingredients and blend on medium speed or until smooth.
2. Pour into serving glass and enjoy the taste.

Nutritional Information

- Preparation Time: 10 minutes
- Servings per Recipe: 2
- Calories: 441
- Protein: 15.1g

- Fat: 12.2g
- Carbohydrates: 24g

Benefits

- Plums fight obesity and best for diabetic patience's (reduces triglyceride and glucose in the body)
- Chia seeds help to boost your metabolism
- Almond provide healthy fat for heart
- Strawberry acts like immune booster

Recipe 25: Strawberry Blast Smoothie

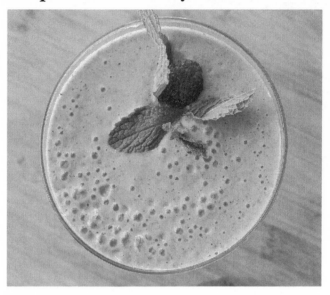

Ingredients

- Cinnamon 1 tsp.
- Dates 5 pieces
- Black grapes 4 oz.
- Apricot 2 oz.
- Almond milk 1 cup
- Cashew powder 2 tbsp.

Preparation Method

1. In a blender, place all ingredients and blend on medium speed or until smooth.
2. Pour into serving glass and enjoy the taste.

Nutritional Information

- Preparation Time: 10 minutes
- Servings per Recipe: 1
- Calories: 301
- Protein: 8.9g
- Fat: 9g

- Carbohydrates: 20.4g

Benefits

- Cinnamon helps to lose weight faster
- Grapes helps to boost the immune system
- Dates helps to reduce weight
- Apricot is rich in vitamins and minerals. Helps to get relief from earaches
- Cashew reduce the risk of developing gallstones

Recipe 26: Papaya Chia Smoothie

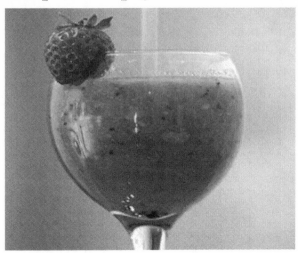

Ingredients

- Chia seeds 1 tbsp.
- Papaya 2 oz.
- Strawberries 2 oz.
- Almond milk 1 cup
- Thyme 2 tbsp.
- Grape fruit ½ piece

Preparation Method

1. In a blender, place all ingredients and blend on medium speed or until smooth.
2. Pour into serving glass and enjoy the taste.

Nutritional Information

- Preparation Time: 10 minutes
- Servings per Recipe: 2
- Calories: 233
- Protein: 4.1g
- Fat: 1.5g
- Carbohydrates: 19.7g

Benefits

- Chia seeds help to boost your metabolism
- Papaya helps to prevent infections (kills intestine worms) and relieves toothache
- Grapefruit Lowers Cholesterol in the body
- Thyme is a natural remedy for bronchitis and cough
- Strawberry acts like immune booster

CHAPTER 7: 26 MOUTHWATERING VEGETABLE SMOOTHIES

Recipe 1: Floret Vegetable Smoothie

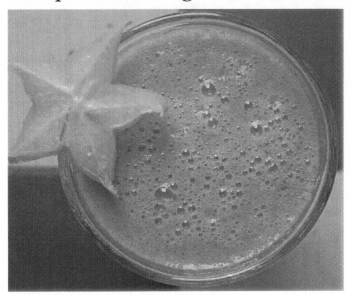

Ingredients

- Water 1 cup
- Half orange
- Baby carrots ¼ cup
- Cauliflower florets ¼ cup
- Broccoli florets ¼ cup
- Celery 1 stalk
- Lemon juice 1 tbsp.
- Dates1
- Chia seeds 1 tbsp.

Preparation Method

1. In a blender, place all ingredients and blend on medium speed or until smooth.
2. Pour into serving glass and enjoy the taste.

Nutritional Information

- Preparation Time: 10 minutes
- Servings per Recipe: 2
- Calories: 199
- Protein: 5.5g
- Fat: 3g
- Carbohydrates: 43.6g

Benefits

- Orange protect the skin from radical damage
- Celery minerals helps to maintain elasticity of the skin
- Chia seeds help to boost your metabolism
- Broccoli helps to increase energy and decrease weight
- Carrot helps to reduce toxicity of the blood (effective on acne)
- Cauliflower is good source of choline, which helps to improve brain health

Recipe 2: Super Green Smoothie

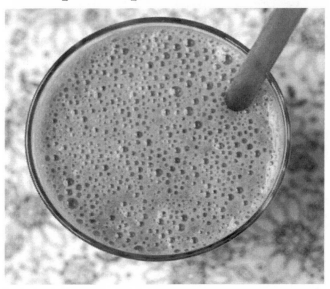

Ingredients

- Kale 1 ½ cup
- Carrots 3 oz.
- Chopped celery 3 oz.
- Orange juice 1 cup
- Parsley 2 oz.
- Fresh Mint 2 oz.

Preparation Method

1. In a blender, place all ingredients and blend on medium speed or until smooth.
2. Pour into serving glass and enjoy the taste.

Nutritional Information

- Preparation Time: 10 minutes
- Servings per Recipe: 2
- Calories: 177
- Protein: 3.2g
- Fat: 5g

- Carbohydrates: 18.1g

Benefits

- Kale are stuffed with vitamins helps in premature aging
- Carrot helps to reduce toxicity of the blood (effective on acne)
- Parsley helps to prevent gas and bloating
- Mint is a great palate cleanser, promotes effective digestion

Recipe 3: Super Weight Loss Shake

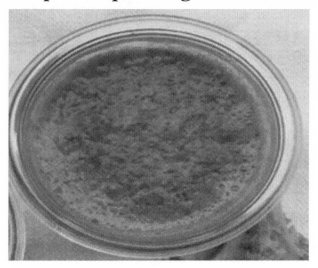

Ingredients

- Spinach 4 oz.
- Mint 1 oz.
- Almond paste 1 ½ tbsp.
- Cucumber 2.5 oz.
- Vanilla 1 tsp.
- Almond milk 1 cup

Preparation Method

1. In a blender, place all ingredients and blend on medium speed or until smooth.
2. Pour into serving glass and enjoy the taste.

Nutritional Information

- Preparation Time: 5 minutes
- Servings per Recipe: 2
- Calories: 229
- Protein: 6.1g
- Fat: 6g
- Carbohydrates: 26g

Benefits

- Spinach restores energy and increase vitality
- Mint is good for digestion, memory loss and prevent pimples
- Almond provide healthy fat for heart
- Cucumber acts like a natural hydrating agent
- Vanilla protects your body from harmful components, such as free radicals and toxins.

Recipe 4: Detox Green Smoothie

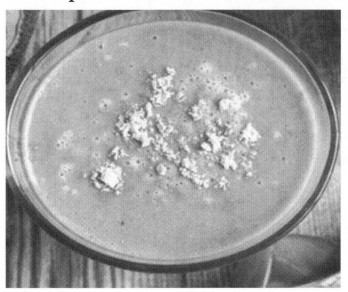

Ingredients

- Spinach 3 oz.
- Kale 4 oz.
- Turmeric 1 tsp.
- Grapes 10
- Celery 2 oz.
- Pumpkin 2 oz.
- Water 1 ½ cup

Preparation Method

1. In a blender, place all ingredients and blend on medium speed or until smooth.
2. Pour into serving glass and enjoy the taste.

Nutritional Information

- Preparation Time: 10 minutes
- Servings per Recipe: 2
- Calories: 256
- Protein: 10g

- Fat: 1.7g
- Carbohydrates: 22g

Benefits

- Turmeric for liver detoxification support
- Pumpkin promotes good vision and lowers blood pressure
- Grapes helps to boost the immune system
- Kale are stuffed with vitamins helps in premature aging
- Spinach leaf membranes contain "thylakoids", boost weight loss by almost 43 percent and stops food cravings for a long time

Recipe 5: Cabbi Root Smoothie

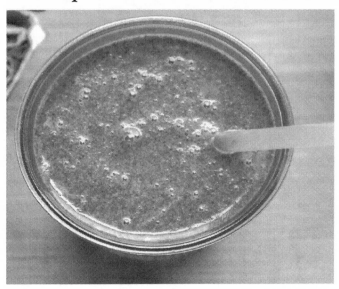

Ingredients

- Beets 3.5 oz.
- Cabbage 3 oz.
- Lemon juice ½ cup
- Nutmeg ¼ tsp.
- Water 1 cup

Preparation Method

1. In a blender, place all ingredients and blend on medium speed or until smooth.
2. Pour into serving glass and enjoy the taste.

Nutritional Information

- Preparation Time: 5 minutes
- Servings per Recipe: 2
- Calories: 199
- Protein: 3.2g
- Fat: 0.9g
- Carbohydrates: 12.2g

Benefits

- Cabbage antioxidants partly responsible for cancer prevention
- Lemon helps to lose weight
- Beets helps to cleanse the blood and strengthen the gall bladder
- Nutmeg provides relief from insomnia and helps to dissolve kidney stones

Recipe 6: Peninsula Ginger Smoothie

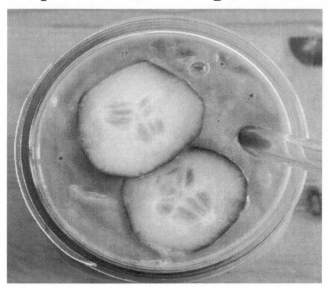

Ingredients

- Baby kale 1 ½ cup
- Beets 2 oz.
- Cucumber 2.5 oz.
- Half asparagus piece
- Ginger 1 oz.
- Hemp seeds 1 tbsp.
- Coconut water 1 cup

Preparation Method

1. In a blender, place all ingredients and blend on medium speed or until smooth.
2. Pour into serving glass and enjoy the taste.

Nutritional Information

- Preparation Time: 10 minutes
- Servings per Recipe: 2
- Calories: 345
- Protein: 12.8g

- Fat: 7.8g
- Carbohydrates: 23g

Benefits

- Cucumber acts like a natural hydrating agent
- Beets helps to cleanse the blood and strengthen the gall bladder
- Asparagus is a brain booster prevents cell damage
- Hemp seeds help to reduce cholesterol and blood pressure
- Ginger acts like metabolic stimulator

Recipe 7: Carrot Cleansing Smoothie

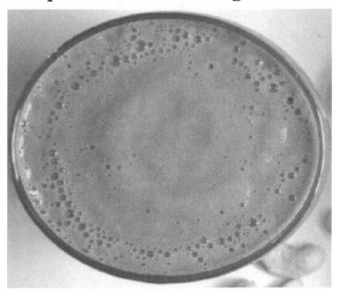

Ingredients

- Butternut squash 1 ½ cup
- Carrot 3 oz.
- Ginger 1 oz.
- Yam 3.5 oz.
- Mint 1 leaf
- Pumpkin seeds 1 tbsp.
- Coconut milk 3 oz.
- Almond milk 2 tbsp.

Preparation Method

- In a blender, place all ingredients and blend on medium speed or until smooth.
- Pour into serving glass and enjoy the taste.

Nutritional Information

- Preparation Time: 10 minutes
- Servings per Recipe: 2
- Calories: 468

- Protein: 26.1g
- Fat: 13g
- Carbohydrates: 31g

Benefits

- Butternut squash prevents high blood pressure and improves eyesight
- Carrot helps to reduce toxicity of the blood (effective on acne)
- Yam helps to heal skin diseases and cures respiratory problems
- Pumpkin seeds improves insulin levels and help to prevent diabetic complications by decreasing oxidative stress in the body
- Mint is a great palate cleanser, promotes effective digestion

Recipe 8: Cinnamon Rabi Smoothie

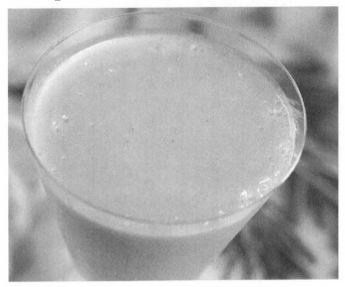

Ingredients

- Kohlrabi 1
- Cinnamon 1 tsp.
- Lemon juice 1 oz.
- Rosemary 1 ½ tbsp.
- Celery 2 oz.
- Parsley 1 tbsp.
- Flax seeds 1 tbsp.
- Ice cubes 3
- Water 1 cup

Preparation Method

1. In a blender, place all ingredients and blend on medium speed or until smooth.
2. Pour into serving glass and enjoy the taste.

Nutritional Information

- Preparation Time: 10 minutes
- Servings per Recipe: 2

- Calories: 177.4
- Protein: 5.1g
- Fat: 3.2g
- Carbohydrates: 31g

Benefits

- Kohlrabi boosts energy levels in body and helps to reduce weight
- Rosemary enhances memory concentration and prevents brain aging
- Parsley helps to prevent gas and bloating
- Celery fights free radicals

Recipe 9: Wheatgrass Detox Smoothie

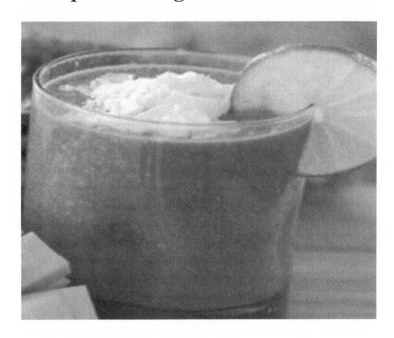

Ingredients

- Spinach 1 oz.
- Wheatgrass 1 oz.
- Turnips 4 oz.
- Sprouts 3 oz.
- Unsweetened coconut flakes 1 ½ oz.
- Coconut water (to max line)

Preparation Method

1. In a blender, place all ingredients and blend on medium speed or until smooth.
2. Pour into serving glass and enjoy the taste.

Nutritional Information

- Preparation Time: 10 minutes
- Servings per Recipe: 2
- Calories: 166

- Protein: 4.5g
- Fat: 3.3g
- Carbohydrates: 22g

Benefits

- Wheatgrass washes drug deposits from the body
- Turnip help to reduce the amount of oxygen needed during exercise and enhance athletic performance
- Sprouts will boost metabolism and prevent anemia
- Coconut flakes might lower your risk of heart disease, diabetes

Recipe 10: Liver Cleansing Smoothie

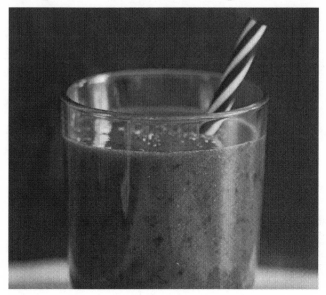

Ingredients

- Dandelion greens 3.5 oz.
- Purple cabbage 1.5 oz.
- Beets 3.5 oz.
- Carrot 2 oz.
- Lemon 1 oz.
- Apple 1 oz.
- Water (to max line)

Preparation Method

1. In a blender, place all ingredients and blend on medium speed or until smooth.
2. Pour into serving glass and enjoy the taste.

Nutritional Information

- Preparation Time: 10 minutes
- Servings per Recipe: 2
- Calories: 144
- Protein: 1g

- Fat: 4g
- Carbohydrates: 24.1g

Benefits

- Dandelion Greens support kidney functionalities and liver cleanser
- Cabbage antioxidants partly responsible for cancer prevention
- Beets helps to cleanse the blood and strengthen the gall bladder
- Carrot helps to reduce toxicity of the blood (effective on acne)

Recipe 11: Sea Ginger Smoothie

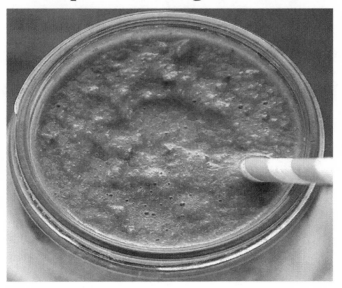

Ingredients

- Ginger root 1 oz.
- Cinnamon 1 tbsp.
- Seaweeds 2 oz.
- Water 1 cup

Preparation Method

1. In a blender, place all ingredients and blend on medium speed or until smooth.
2. Pour into serving glass and enjoy the taste.

Nutritional Information

- Preparation Time: 10 minutes
- Servings per Recipe: 1
- Calories: 87
- Protein: 3g
- Fat: 0.6g
- Carbohydrates: 9g

Benefits

- Ginger acts like metabolic stimulator
- Seaweed provides daily dose of iodine and metabolize fats for energy
- cinnamon helps to lose weight faster

Recipe 12: Extreme Detox Smoothie

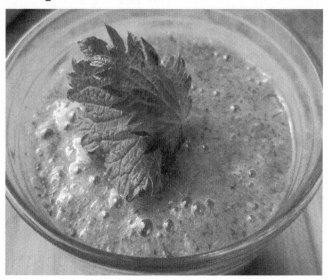

Ingredients

- Carrot 3 oz.
- Pear 2 oz.
- Endive 2 oz.
- Broccoli florets 3.5 oz.
- Water 1 cup

Preparation Method

1. In a blender, place all ingredients and blend on medium speed or until smooth.
2. Pour into serving glass and enjoy the taste.

Nutritional Information

- Preparation Time: 5 minutes
- Servings per Recipe: 2
- Calories: 142
- Protein: 4.8g
- Fat: 0.95g
- Carbohydrates: 19g

Benefits

- Pears are natural boost of energy because of its glucose and fructose
- Endives protect lungs and maintain healthy mucous membranes
- Broccoli helps to increase energy and decrease weight
- Carrot helps to reduce toxicity of the blood (effective on acne)

Recipe 13: Yoga Cleanse Smoothie

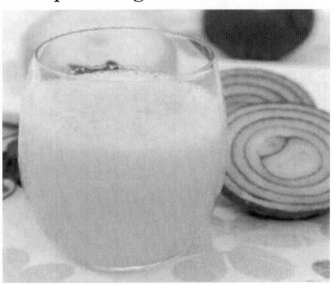

Ingredients

- Onions 3
- Banana 1
- Basil 2 tsp.
- Water ½ cup
- Cloves 1 tsp.

Preparation Method

1. In a blender, place all ingredients and blend on medium speed or until smooth.
2. Pour into serving glass and enjoy the taste.

Nutritional Information

- Preparation Time: 10 minutes
- Servings per Recipe: 1
- Calories: 172
- Protein: 5.6g
- Fat: 1.1g
- Carbohydrates: 10g

Benefits

- Onions reduces risk of gastric ulcers and immediate relief from burning sensation
- Cloves prevent specific bacteria spread cholera
- Basil prevent oxygen based damages
- Banana reduces risk of heart diseases

Recipe 14: Creamy Zucchini Smoothie

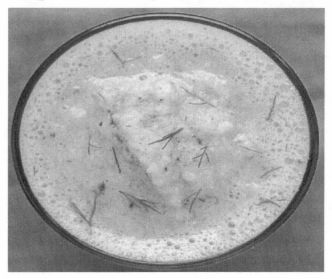

Ingredients

- Zucchini 2
- Tomato 1
- Red onion 1
- Dill 6 springs
- Sweet Potatoes 2 oz.

Preparation Method

1. In a blender, place all ingredients and blend on medium speed or until smooth.
2. Pour into serving glass and enjoy the taste.

Nutritional Information

- Preparation Time: 10 minutes
- Servings per Recipe: 1
- Calories: 151
- Protein: 6.1g
- Fat: 4.5g
- Carbohydrates: 28g

Benefits

- Zucchini prevents cancer and cardiovascular diseases
- Tomatoes improves skin's ability to protect against UV rays
- Dill reduces menstrual cramps and depression
- Sweet potato improves red and white blood cells production

Recipe 15: Swiss Greens Smoothie

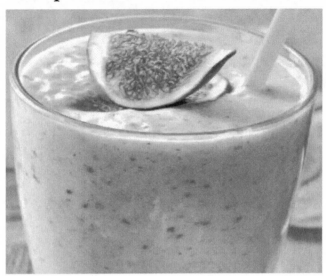

Ingredients

- Swiss collard 3.5 oz.
- Choy sum 2 oz.
- Radish leafs 2 oz.
- Fresh fig 3.5 oz.
- Black pepper 3g

Preparation Method

1. In a blender, place all ingredients and blend on medium speed or until smooth.
2. Pour into serving glass and enjoy the taste.

Nutritional Information

- Preparation Time: 8 minutes
- Servings per Recipe: 2
- Calories: 192
- Protein: 5.1g
- Fat: 1.7g
- Carbohydrates: 23.2g

Benefits

- Swiss collard, due to his phytonutrient antioxidants, it acts an anti-inflammatory agent
- Choy sum develops resistance against pro-inflammatory free radicals
- Fig helps to control blood pressure
- Pepper helps in hormone balance

Recipe 16: Celery Seeds Smoothie

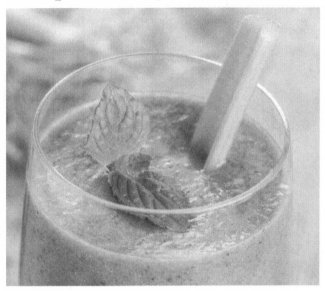

Ingredients

- Celery 1 cup
- Ground chia seeds 2 tsp.
- Parsley ½ cup
- Chicory 1 oz.
- Ground Ceylon cinnamon 1 tsp.

Preparation Method

1. In a blender, place all ingredients and blend on medium speed or until smooth.
2. Pour into serving glass and enjoy the taste.

Nutritional Information

- Preparation Time: 8 minutes
- Servings per Recipe: 1
- Calories: 166
- Protein: 5.9g
- Fat: 3.5g
- Carbohydrates: 19.9g

Benefits

- Celery helps to reduce high blood pressure
- Chia seeds help to boost your metabolism
- Parsley is an immune booster
- Chicory helps to relieves constipation and aids gut health
- Cinnamon helps to lose weight faster

Recipe 17: Clove Cress Smoothie

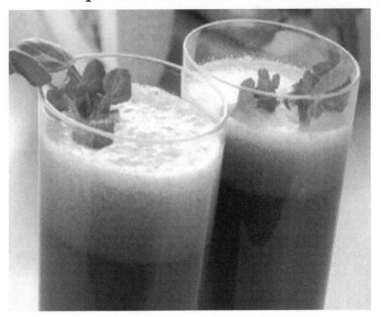

Ingredients

- Cloves 1 tbsp.
- Watercress 1 ½ cup
- Wheat grass 1 tbsp.
- Kale 2 oz.
- Cayenne pepper 1 tsp.

Preparation Method

1. In a blender, place all ingredients and blend on medium speed or until smooth.
2. Pour into serving glass and enjoy the taste.

Nutritional Information

- Preparation Time: 8 minutes
- Servings per Recipe: 1
- Calories: 176
- Protein: 12.2g
- Fat: 3.3g

- Carbohydrates: 17g

Benefits

- Cloves prevent specific bacteria spread cholera
- Watercress help to boost immunity and thyroid prevention
- Wheat grass helps to neutralize toxins and environmental pollutants in the body
- Kale helps to counteract oxidative damage by free radicals in the body

Recipe 18: Asparagus Melon Smoothie

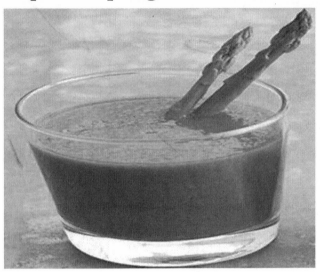

Ingredients

- Asparagus 6 oz.
- Watermelon 5 oz.
- Mint 2 oz.
- Cucumber 3 oz.
- Fennel seeds 1 tsp.
- Ice cube 1

Preparation Method

1. In a blender, place all ingredients and blend on medium speed or until smooth.
2. Pour into serving glass and enjoy the taste.

Nutritional Information

- Preparation Time: 10 minutes
- Servings per Recipe: 3
- Calories: 156
- Protein: 2.25g
- Fat: 2g
- Carbohydrates: 18g

Benefits

- Asparagus is a brain booster prevents cell damage
- Watermelon works as a natural viagra, which relaxes and dilates blood vessels in the body
- Mint is good for digestion, memory loss and prevent pimples
- Fennel seeds is home remedy for flatulence and indigestion

Recipe 19: Coco Vera Smoothie

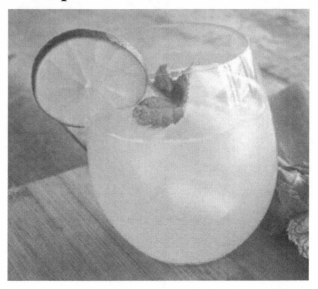

Ingredients

- Coconut water 3 oz.
- Aloe vera 3 oz.
- Crookneck squash 3 oz.
- Garlic juice 1 oz.

Preparation Method

1. In a blender, place all ingredients and blend on medium speed or until smooth.
2. Pour into serving glass and enjoy the taste.

Nutritional Information

- Preparation Time: 5 minutes
- Servings per Recipe: 2
- Calories: 190
- Protein: 4.1g
- Fat: 0.6g
- Carbohydrates: 10g

Benefits

- Aloe Vera repairs damaged or torn vaginal walls
- Coconut water balances the electrolytes in the body which improves blood circulation and muscle function
- Crookneck squash fights infections and supports for better immune system
- Garlic helps to reduce cholesterol levels and risk of heart diseases. Additionally, it will block tumors by slowing DNA replication

Recipe 20: Horse Beets Smoothie

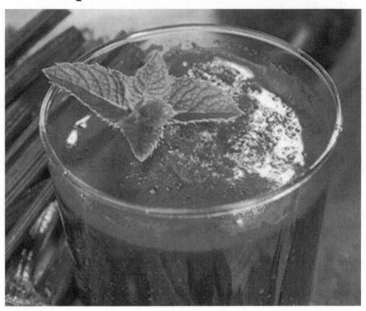

Ingredients

- Beets 6 oz.
- Ground horseradish 2 tbsp.
- Parsley 2 oz.
- Garlic 1 oz.
- Ginger 1 oz.

Preparation Method

1. In a blender, place all ingredients and blend on medium speed or until smooth.
2. Pour into serving glass and enjoy the taste.

Nutritional Information

- Preparation Time: 5 minutes
- Servings per Recipe: 2
- Calories: 213
- Protein: 8g
- Fat: 1.5g

- Carbohydrates: 17g

Benefits

- Beets helps to cleanse the blood and strengthen the gall bladder
- Horseradish aids in weight loss, stimulates urination and eliminates risks of tube defects
- Garlic helps to reduce cholesterol levels and risk of heart diseases. Additionally, it will block tumors by slowing DNA replication
- Ginger acts like metabolic stimulator

Recipe 21: Fennel Chives Smoothie

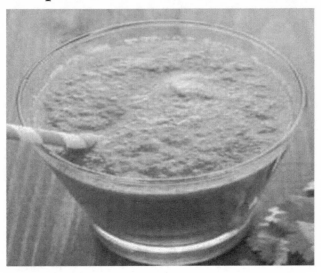

Ingredients

- Ground fennel seeds 2.5 oz.
- Cilantro 1 cup
- Chives 1 cup
- Turmeric 1 tsp.
- Acorn squash 2 oz.

Preparation Method

1. In a blender, place all ingredients and blend on medium speed or until smooth.
2. Pour into serving glass and enjoy the taste.

Nutritional Information

- Preparation Time: 8 minutes
- Servings per Recipe: 2
- Calories: 166
- Protein: 9g
- Fat: 2.4g
- Carbohydrates: 20.4g

Benefits

- Fennel seeds is home remedy for flatulence and indigestion
- Cilantro helps to build strong bones and also known as anti-diabetic plant
- Turmeric for liver detoxification support
- Chives helps to lower the stomach cancer and improves bone health
- Acorn squash aids in eliminating constipation, diarrhea, cramping and bloating

Recipe 22: Hawthorn Nettle Smoothie

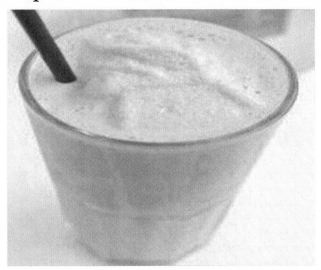

Ingredients

- Nettle leaf 1 cup
- Hawthorn 2.5 oz.
- Wheat grass 1 tbsp.
- Cayenne pepper 5.3g
- Walnuts 5

Preparation Method

1. In a blender, place all ingredients and blend on medium speed or until smooth.
2. Pour into serving glass and enjoy the taste.

Nutritional Information

- Preparation Time: 5 minutes
- Servings per Recipe: 1
- Calories: 257
- Protein: 10.6g
- Fat: 2g
- Carbohydrates: 14g

Benefits

- Nettle leaf prevents eczema and stimulate contraction in pregnant women's
- Wheatgrass washes drug deposits from the body
- Cayenne pepper helps in hormone balance
- Hawthorn increase the transmission of nerve signals in the body

Recipe 23: Artichoke Greens Smoothie

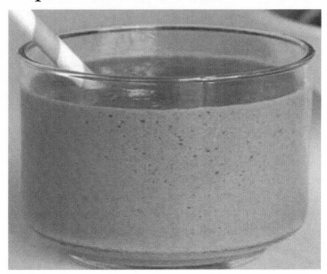

Ingredients

- Artichoke 3 oz.
- Cabbage 3 oz.
- Basil 2.5 oz.
- Jicama 2.5 oz.
- Carrot 2 oz.
- Turmeric ½ tsp.

Preparation Method

1. In a blender, place all ingredients and blend on medium speed or until smooth.
2. Pour into serving glass and enjoy the taste.

Nutritional Information

- Preparation Time: 10 minutes
- Servings per Recipe: 1
- Calories: 181
- Protein: 9.1g
- Fat: 1.5g
- Carbohydrates: 16.6g

Benefits

- Cabbage antioxidants partly responsible for cancer prevention
- Basil prevent oxygen based damages
- Jicama helps to increase bone strength and functionalities of brain
- Turmeric for liver detoxification support
- Artichoke improves brain, cognitive and liver health

Recipe 24: Summer Yellow Smoothie

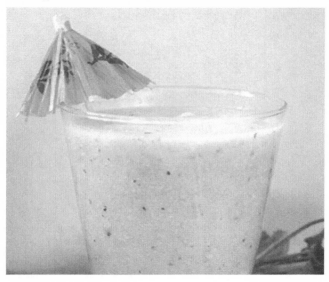

Ingredients

- Yellow summer squash5 oz.
- Asparagus 5 oz.
- Celery 2.5 oz.
- Mint 2 oz.
- Garlic 4 tsp.

Preparation Method

1. In a blender, place all ingredients and blend on medium speed or until smooth.
2. Pour into serving glass and enjoy the taste.

Nutritional Information

- Preparation Time: 5 minutes
- Servings per Recipe: 2
- Calories: 167
- Protein: 3.1g
- Fat: 4.2g
- Carbohydrates: 19g

Benefits

- Squash aids in eliminating constipation, diarrhea, cramping and bloating
- Asparagus is a brain booster prevents cell damage
- Mint is good for digestion, memory loss and prevent pimples
- Garlic helps to reduce cholesterol levels and risk of heart diseases. Additionally, it will block tumors by slowing DNA replication

Recipe 25: Pepper Chives Smoothie

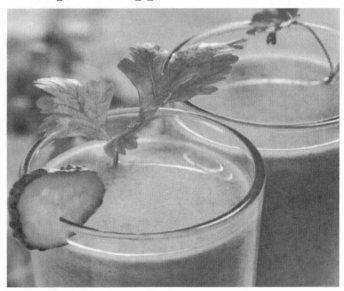

Ingredients

- Cayenne pepper ½ tsp.
- Chives 1 cup
- Coriander leaves 2.5 oz.
- Nettle leaf 1.5 oz.
- Artichoke 1.5 oz.
- Wheatgrass 1 tbsp.

Preparation Method

1. In a blender, place all ingredients and blend on medium speed or until smooth.
2. Pour into serving glass and enjoy the taste.

Nutritional Information

- Preparation Time: 10 minutes
- Servings per Recipe: 1
- Calories: 234
- Protein: 11g
- Fat: 2.4g

- Carbohydrates: 21g

Benefits

- Artichoke improves brain, cognitive and liver health
- Wheatgrass washes drug deposits from the body
- Nettle leaf prevents eczema and stimulate contraction in pregnant women's
- Chives helps to lower the stomach cancer and improves bone health
- Cayenne pepper helps in hormone balance

Recipe 26: Beet Carrot Smoothie

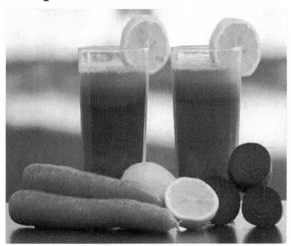

Ingredients

- Carrot 2 oz.
- Beets 2 oz.
- Fresh mint 1 oz.
- Lemon juice 2 tbsp.
- Fresh ginger 1 tbsp.
- Star anise 1

Preparation Method

1. In a blender, place all ingredients and blend on medium speed or until smooth.
2. Pour into serving glass and enjoy the taste.

Nutritional Information

- Preparation Time: 10 minutes
- Servings per Recipe: 1
- Calories: 198
- Protein: 3.3g
- Fat: 1g
- Carbohydrates: 16g

Benefits

- Beets helps to cleanse the blood and strengthen the gall bladder
- Carrot helps to reduce toxicity of the blood (effective on acne)
- Mint is a great palate cleanser, promotes effective digestion
- Ginger produces sexual arousal, which increases stimulation in the brain
- Star anise will be used as anti-fungal, anti-bacterial and for influenza

Conclusion

The information provided in this book will help you to educate in the right way toward your successful ambition to follow paleo lifestyle and maintain good health throughout your life. Before you start each day, remember and remind yourself about wonderful benefits you achieve while the following paleo diet and tell yourself that you can do this for improving your health and a better environment. Once again thank you for downloading our book and we hope you will achieve your dreams.

--- Sarah Moore

Made in the USA
Lexington, KY
23 April 2019